University
information services

Transitions
in Care

Meeting the Challenges
of Type 1 Diabetes
in Young Adults

Howard A. Wolpert, MD
Barbara J. Anderson, PhD
Jill Weissberg-Benchell, PhD, CDE

American

Director, Book Publishing, John Fedor; *Managing Editor, Book Publishing,* Abraham Ogden; *Editor,* Greg Guthrie; *Production Manager and Composition,* Melissa Sprott; *Cover Design,* Koncept, Inc.; *Printer,* United Graphics, Inc.

Printed in the United States of America
1 3 5 7 9 10 8 6 4 2

The suggestions and information contained in this publication are generally consistent with the *Clinical Practice Recommendations* and other policies of the American Diabetes Association, but they do not represent the policy or position of the Association or any of its boards or committees. Reasonable steps have been taken to ensure the accuracy of the information presented. However, the American Diabetes Association cannot ensure the safety or efficacy of any product or service described in this publication. Individuals are advised to consult a physician or other appropriate health care professional before undertaking any diet or exercise program or taking any medication referred to in this publication. Professionals must use and apply their own professional judgment, experience, and training and should not rely solely on the information contained in this publication before prescribing any diet, exercise, or medication. The American Diabetes Association—its officers, directors, employees, volunteers, and members—assumes no responsibility or liability for personal or other injury, loss, or damage that may result from the suggestions or information in this publication.

♾ The paper in this publication meets the requirements of the ANSI Standard Z39.48-1992 (permanence of paper).

ADA titles may be purchased for business or promotional use or for special sales. To purchase this book in large quantities, or for custom editions of this book with your logo, contact Lee Romano Sequeira, Special Sales & Promotions, at the address below, or at LRomano@diabetes.org or call 703-299-2046.

American Diabetes Association
1701 North Beauregard Street
Alexandria, Virginia 22311

Library of Congress Cataloging-in-Publication Data
Wolpert, Howard A., 1958-
  Transitions in care : a guide to the challenges of type 1 diabetes in young adults / Howard A. Wolpert, Barbara J. Anderson, Jill Weissberg-Benchell.
     p. ; cm.
  Includes index.
  ISBN 1-58040-172-4 (alk. paper)
  1. Diabetes in children. 2. Young adults--Health and hygiene. 3. Patient education.
  [DNLM: 1. Diabetes Mellitus, Type 1. 2. Adolescent. WK 810 W866t 2006] I.
Anderson, Barbara J. (Barbara Jane), 1947- II. Weissberg-Benchell, Jill. III. American Diabetes Association. IV. Title.

  RJ420.D5W65 2006
  618.92'462--dc22

                              2005035421

Contents

Why We Wrote This Book

Almost anyone who has cared for someone in their late teens and twenties, either through parenting or treatment, knows that this is a unique and distinct phase of life. These are times filled with the tasks that map out the course of a life: the engrossing search for self and one's place in society, the first steps toward career and financial independence, and deepening emotional involvements. The young adult is no longer an adolescent, but frequently is not yet completely independent from family support either. This is also a time of life when the person with type 1 diabetes assumes full responsibility for his or her own diabetes care and a period when the earliest signs of diabetes complications will often first present. The initiation of intensive therapy during this phase, when lifelong patterns of self-care behavior are being set, can have a significant impact on an individual's risk for future complications. Intensive insulin therapy requires discipline and sacrifice, not to mention responsibility and adequate support. Clearly, for the young adult who faces many competing demands for his or her time and attention, diabetes self-care may not always be a priority.

The diabetes clinician needs to be aware that any perceived reluctance to intensify therapy on the part of the young-adult patient may be because his or her focus is naturally drawn to the competing demands of education, relationships, and career building. A successful relationship will be founded in a long-term view of care, focusing primarily on a directly collaborative partnership that ensures that the young adult remains actively involved in his or her own health care. Clinicians can jumpstart this process by envisioning their primary role as an agent for behavioral change. The clinician's role should resemble that of a *coach* (who equips young adults with the skills needed to manage their diabetes) and a *guide* (who helps young adults make informed decisions about living with diabetes and works with the patient in developing a plan aimed at reaching optimal diabetes control). A priority in care is to ensure that patients remain invested in their self-care behaviors and engage in active problem solving. Young adults who have these tools are less likely to fall into the trap of frustration, hopelessness, and disengagement from medical follow-up.

We have found that the needs of young adults with diabetes fall outside of the traditional focus of both adult and pediatric medicine, which is the reason for this book. Our clinical experience has taught us of the need for a thoughtful, systematic approach to assist young adults in their transition to healthy adulthood. In this book, we offer a framework for thinking about the important issues in diabetes care for young adults. The first section provides background information on the young-adult period with which young adults with diabetes, their parents, and care providers should be familiar.

Following that, the book is written in two voices. One voice, introduced in the second section and directed to young adults and their families and friends, focuses on the challenges and demands of living with diabetes and presents guidance in making informed decisions about diabetes during this complex phase of life. The other voice, arising in the third section, provides a perspective of how the complexities of this developmental stage affect the health professional's clinical role.

While we have used different voices for each section, this hardly means that each part of the book is exclusive to that audience. We strongly encourage you, whether you are a young adult, parent, or care provider, to cover all of this material. Knowledge, particularly when concerning diabetes, is one of the most important tools in optimizing care, especially for a patient group that has been largely overlooked in clinical history.

Howard A. Wolpert, MD
Joslin Diabetes Center, Boston, MA

Barbara J. Anderson, PhD
Baylor College of Medicine, Houston, TX

Jill Weissberg-Benchell, PhD, CDE
Children's Memorial Hospital, Chicago, IL

1

For All of Us:
The Challenges of Young Adulthood

DEVELOPMENT OF THE EMERGING ADULT

In contrast to the views of traditional developmental psychology, recent developmental theorists subdivide the young-adult period into two phases: *1)* an early phase corresponding to the years after high school (~18–22 years old) and *2)* a later phase when more traditional adult roles are assumed (~23–30 years old). This age division is more or less arbitrary and may not apply to all individuals, and not all individuals or cultures progress through the young-adult period according to these two phases. However, thinking about young adulthood as consisting of two phases provides a valuable framework in which to approach care for this specific age-group. Viewing young adults from this perspective can help ensure that the parents' attention and the clinician's approach and focus are matched to the young adult's life circumstances and readiness to become an active participant in diabetes management.

The First Phase of the Young-Adult Period

Levinson and colleagues and Arnett theorized that, among U.S. young adults, the developmental tasks just after high school do not frequently mesh with the expectations of the various institutions responsible for them. Specifically, this describes a difference in point of view concerning what traits young adults feel they need to develop to become adults and which traits institutions expect their young adults to already have.

Arnett asked individuals between the ages of 18 and 24 years what attributes made someone an adult. Four specific achievements were cited:

1. The ability to accept responsibility for oneself.

2. The ability to make independent decisions.

3. The ability to become financially independent.

4. The ability to independently form one's own beliefs and values.

Interestingly, most of the young adults interviewed did not believe that they had achieved these goals. In fact, most young people in the U.S. do not believe that they have achieved these goals until they are in their late twenties. Several dilemmas confront young adults in the first phase of the young-adult period. This phase is characterized by the desire for, yet simultaneous fear of, independence. Freedom from parental supervision comes with responsibilities that can be daunting. The young adult begins to face issues such as how to find and keep a place to live, pay bills, balance a checkbook, manage credit, begin or sustain potentially long-term relationships, and choose and maintain a career. While young adults are trying to balance all of these new freedoms and responsibilities, they will likely do so with less help from their parents and less structure in their daily routine. In addition, when young adults move away from their hometown, as is common, they make these decisions in a place where few people know them and where their closest friends are far away.

Similarly, the family of a young adult with type 1 diabetes faces several dilemmas. Here are some of the issues that families must begin addressing.

- Whether the young adult and the parents will tolerate separation and increasing independence and still remain connected.

- Whether the parents could possibly become overinvolved or cut off relationships prematurely.

- How the young adult copes with the potential of remaining dependent on his or her parents for both tangible support, such as money and housing, and emotional support as he or she develops into an adult.

- The parents' ability to treat their older children as adults with their own separate, independent lives.

- How the parent copes with the often-difficult transition from a hands-on role in caring for a child to becoming a consultant for his or her young-adult child. Parents must also consider how they will handle the shift from direct interaction with their child's physician or nurse to relying on secondhand information from the young adult.

To place these dilemmas in perspective, the data from the 2000 U.S. Census tell us that 56% of men and 43% of women between the ages of 18 and 24 years still live at home with their parents. For those who don't live at home, 30% of men and 35% of women live with roommates. In fact, only 4% of individuals in this age-group live alone. Therefore, the assumption that individuals in this age-group are independent tends to be misrepresented, both in terms of adult development and in regard to where they live.

During the first phase of young adulthood, which has been called the "early adult transition," the person may be shifting geographically, economically, and emotionally away from the parental home. Furthermore, if the 18- to 22-year-old has also gone to a college or trade school, then his or her new life will be marked by additional changes, distractions, and demands. For most young adults, these competing educational, economic, and social priorities detract from a focused commitment to chronic-disease management. Even though young adults face these competing demands on a day-to-day basis, most do not believe that they have all of the skills necessary to remain independent. Therefore, it may be unrealistic to expect young adults with diabetes in this phase to intensify their glycemic control, learn pump therapy, or begin a new relationship with an adult-care provider. Furthermore, the first phase is often marked by feelings of invulnerability and a tendency to reject adult control. For obvious reasons, this further limits a young adult's receptiveness to change.

The young adult's duration of diabetes can be an important factor in the transition of the young adult to independent self-management. For some young adults who have had diabetes since childhood, it is important to explore formative diabetes experiences. Longitudinal studies of pediatric patients with type 1 diabetes in the U.K. and U.S. have reported that behavior problems during the adolescent years clearly predict emotional and physical health complications in the young-adult period. The young adult who previously encountered unrealistic expectations of diabetes management and who has had a legacy of punitive and judgmental medical encounters is especially vulnerable to *diabetes burnout,* a condition characterized by feelings of inadequacy or guilt from chronically failing at diabetes management. If the young adult has had a negative socialization experience growing up with diabetes and does not have a solid, constructive relationship with pediatric providers, early transfer to an adult provider (having some experience with adolescents and young adults with type 1 diabetes) may be in the patient's best interest.

Even for other patients whose prior medical experience has been largely positive and encouraging, continued follow-up with familiar and trusted pediatric providers and educators is likely the most effective course of action. Many young adults feel vulnerable after finishing high school, so delaying the transition to adult care until the distractions and insecurities of this period pass may ensure stronger self-care practices in the future. Prior exposure to the adult provider should help young adults make a smooth transition and minimize loss to medical follow-up.

The "Second Phase" of the Young-Adult Period

During the second phase of the young-adult period (~23–30 years old), the young adult's sense of identity matures. These young adults also assume more "adult-like" roles in society, such as stable intimate relationships and employment. During the second phase, young adults start making plans for their future life and usually demonstrate a growing recognition of the importance of better glycemic control and increased receptiveness to improving self-care behavior. Life partners can be important supporters of and agents for change, and a shared sense of investment in the future will often catalyze this change in self-care behavior. This period—when lifelong patterns of behavior are set—offers a critical window of opportunity for health care education interventions. Health care providers have a crucial role at this stage in preparing and motivating young adults with diabetes to assume self-management responsibilities.

2

For the Young Adult: Preparing for Your Journey

Have you ever been told to get your blood glucose under control? Have you been told that doing this will improve your chances of living a long, complication-free life? Of course you have, and it's true.

Evidence from the Diabetes Control and Complications Trial (DCCT) backs up that claim. The DCCT studied over 1,400 individuals with type 1 diabetes over a 10-year period (1983–1993). The study subjects were randomly divided into two groups: *1)* a "conventional treatment" group that took up to two insulin injections a day (the standard of care at the time) and *2)* an "intensive therapy" group that used multiple daily insulin injections (three or more injections a day) or an insulin pump. Not surprisingly, the intensive therapy group ended up in a lot better shape. In fact, they had less than half as many severe eye, kidney, and nerve complications as those in the conventional group.

But there's more to this. Follow-up studies of the DCCT participants showed that optimal glucose control was still providing some protection against developing complications a decade later, even if that control didn't meet the DCCT's rigorous standards. In short, good blood glucose control, even if it isn't *perfect* control, significantly improves your quality of life now and in the future.

This should underscore the importance of *optimizing* your glucose control, and doing so will be a lifelong goal. Optimizing your blood glucose means that you should do the best you possibly can, because it matters in the end. The challenge comes in deciding *how* you go about achieving good control and *how* you balance the daily demands of diabetes with the other demands of life.

In this section, we will explore this difficult balancing act between diabetes and the rest of your life. In addition, we will outline a road map to help you get and stay on track with your diabetes.

THE BASICS: INSULIN AND TYPE 1 DIABETES

Before we get to the principles about how to achieve good glucose control, we're going to present a brief review of how insulin helps the body use (or metabolize) glucose for energy.

As you probably know, insulin is a hormone produced by the beta cells in the pancreas. The pancreas releases insulin into the bloodstream in two different ways—as basal and bolus insulin. Figure 1 illustrates how insulin and glucose interact in a healthy human over a 24-hour period. Obviously, people with type 1 diabetes have a different insulin action profile.

Figure 1: 24-Hour Insulin and Glucose Profile in a Person Without Diabetes

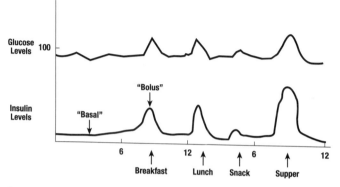

Basal Insulin

The body releases a small amount of insulin all the time. This small dosage is called *background* or *basal* insulin. Basal insulin controls your blood glucose levels between meals and overnight. The body requires this constant insulin release because the liver acts as a glucose "reservoir," continuously releasing glucose to provide energy for basic functions in the body, such as brain activity. Basal insulin keeps this steady release of glucose under control. Without basal insulin, there would be an excessive release of glucose by the liver and glucose levels in the blood would rise. Also, in the absence of basal insulin, the liver starts producing ketone bodies, and these can accumulate in the body, leading to a dangerous condition known as diabetic ketoacidosis.

Bolus Insulin

The body releases large, surging doses of insulin when blood glucose levels rise after eating. This is called *bolus* insulin. Bolus insulin causes the tissues of the body to absorb glucose from the bloodstream. The amount of insulin produced in these mealtime surges is very precisely controlled to ensure that there is just enough to take care of the carbohydrates being eaten. Eat a bit more, and more insulin is produced; eat a bit less, and less insulin is produced.

How This Works in Type 1 Diabetes

In type 1 diabetes, the immune system, which normally combats infections, misguidedly attacks and kills the beta cells in the pancreas. This process happens gradually, but the results are typically the same. Over a period of months or years, the immune system kills most of the pancreatic beta cells. Your beta cells are special cells in the pancreas, called islet cells, that are specifically designed to generate insulin. Without them, the body no longer produces insulin. Therefore, the fundamental challenge in treating type 1 diabetes is replacing the insulin your body no longer makes by taking just enough insulin to match your body's needs.

Approaches to Insulin Treatment

The insulin profile in Figure 2 may be familiar to you. This is the traditional approach to insulin replacement. In this type of insulin therapy, you take injections of bolus insulin, either rapid-acting

(Humalog, NovoLog) or fast-acting (Regular) insulin, at breakfast and dinner. Additional injections of long-acting insulin (usually NPH) provide your body with basal insulin at breakfast and at bedtime. The rapid-acting insulin injections take care of the carbohydrates eaten at breakfast and dinner. Meanwhile, the morning injection of NPH covers lunch, and the evening injection of NPH controls the glucose that the liver releases overnight.

Figure 2: Injection Therapy Using Humalog/Novolog and NPH/Lente

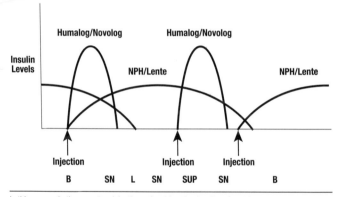

In this approach, there are two injections of rapid-acting insulin at breakfast and dinner and two injections of NPH/Lente insulin to provide the basal insulin.

Optimizing glucose control using this insulin program can be challenging. There are some notable downsides, too.

▪ It forces you to follow a fairly regimented and consistent routine and meal plan. You must eat meals and snacks at specific times, and the carbohydrate content of meals and snacks needs to be nearly the same every day.

- If you eat a late lunch, the morning injection of NPH will kick in and hypoglycemia (low blood glucose) may result.

- You often need to eat between-meal snacks (especially at mid-morning) to prevent the long-acting insulin taken at breakfast from causing hypoglycemia.

- If you eat too many carbohydrates in a meal or snack, then there may be insufficient insulin available and your glucose level will rise. If you eat too few carbohydrates, then there may be more insulin in your body than you need, causing blood glucose levels to fall too low (hypoglycemia).

- You need to wake up at the same time every day. If you sleep in, the longer-acting insulin taken the evening before (to control the production of glucose by the liver overnight) may run out, resulting in increased blood glucose levels (hyperglycemia).

As with most choices in life, there is a trade-off with this type of insulin program. There is no need for a lunchtime injection, which can be an important consideration for someone who would find this extra injection inconvenient or impractical, such as at school or work. But if you want to keep your glucose within any targeted range, you will need to follow a fairly regimented and consistent routine and meal plan. This means that meals and snacks need to be eaten at specific times, and the carbohydrate content of meals needs to be consistent from one day to the next.

The development of peakless long-acting insulins and insulin pumps has presented new options for insulin replacement. With these tools, we can come closer to mimicking the way the beta cells of the pancreas release insulin into the body.

Figure 3: Schematic representation of idealized insulin effect provided by three daily injections with rapid-acting insulin at meals and once-daily insulin glargine at bedtime. B, breakfast; L, lunch; S, supper; HS, bedtime; Arrow, time of insulin injection.

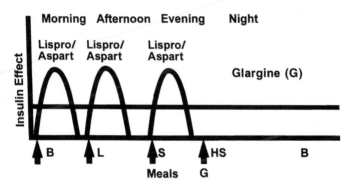

This approach to insulin replacement—also known as *basal-bolus therapy*—allows more flexibility in a person's schedule and eating. Insulin can be matched to cover the amount of food eaten, and there's no need to eat on schedule. In addition, because the longer-acting insulin does not peak, there's no need to eat snacks between meals to prevent hypoglycemia. This can be quite helpful with weight control, but this type of insulin program generally requires more injections or the use of an insulin pump.

WHICH INSULIN PROGRAM IS RIGHT FOR ME?

For many people, different insulin programs fit different phases of life. For example, during the elementary and high school years, taking a lunchtime injection in the cafeteria can be impractical or embarrassing. For people at this stage, the NPH-based insulin program may be the best option. Later, during the college years, the extra flexibility provided by basal-bolus therapy may provide real advantages, especially if your schedule changes from day to day.

There will likely be a time when optimizing your blood glucose levels becomes more of a priority, preferably sooner rather than later. When you're ready to make a long-term commitment to better blood glucose control, there are a couple of considerations to weigh when deciding whether to use injections or a pump for basal-bolus insulin therapy. Some may find it a hassle to take an extra injection every time they want a large snack or have eaten more than planned. An insulin pump makes it convenient to take a bolus of insulin whenever needed. If you are considering using a pump, there are two key questions you need to ask yourself.

- How comfortable will I feel while wearing a pump, which shows everyone that I have diabetes?

- Do I have the time to learn how to correctly use a pump?

The early-adult and college years are often when serious relationships (both romantic and platonic) outside of the family first develop, and some people will find the pump a bit too obvious and public. Some find that it's better to have already dealt with the demands of getting settled into a new job or college before trying the pump. Additionally, some people may feel more comfortable if they "work up" to an insulin pump by learning the ropes with multiple injection therapy. A handy book for people who are thinking about whether the insulin pump is right for them is *Smart Pumping,* by Howard Wolpert.

You alone live with and manage your diabetes day to day, so only you will really know which type of insulin program suits you best. More importantly, only you can know if you are even ready to optimize your glucose control. You make the decisions in caring for your diabetes—this is one of the more enlightening yet intimidating truths about growing up. At this stage in life, your health care team is there to coach and guide you, but from here on out, you make the decisions that affect your life.

THE FUNDAMENTAL SKILLS IN MANAGING DIABETES

By now, you should realize that the key skill in managing your diabetes is *learning to think like a pancreas* by matching insulin doses with carbohydrate intake. So, understanding how insulin acts and determining the carbohydrate content of your foods are the essential elements of effectively managing diabetes.

A comprehensive review of all you need to know to improve your glucose control is beyond the scope of this book. For that, sessions with your health care team, especially a certified diabetes educator (CDE), are the best sources. Here are some of the important skills you will need to master.

■ Understand how rapid- and long-acting insulins act in your body, such as how quickly they start to work, when they peak, and how long they last.

- Learn how to find the carbohydrate and fat content of the foods you eat. Learn to read food labels, judge portion sizes, and use reference lists or books, such as *The Diabetes Carbohydrate and Fat Gram Guide,* by Lea Ann Holzmeister. Keeping a food diary can be helpful.

- Learn how to use blood glucose monitoring to determine your insulin doses.

- Learn how to use the glucose numbers you record in your logbook to identify glucose patterns.

- Learn how to troubleshoot and treat hypoglycemia.

- Learn how to manage your glucose levels before, during, and after exercise.

- Learn how to manage your glucose levels when you become ill.

- Learn how to manage your glucose levels when you drink alcohol.

Learning is an ongoing, lifelong process, and diabetes education is no different. You'll find throughout your life that you never quite stop learning about diabetes or how to better improve your diabetes self-care. For example, if you eat out a lot, you may learn to spot hidden fats in food, which can slow your digestion of carbohydrate and prolong your after-meal glucose rises. If you start doing more of your own cooking, you might learn how to lower the fat content of favorite family recipes or determine its carbohydrate content.

BLOOD GLUCOSE AND YOU

Keeping Perspective on Blood Glucose Goals

Expanding your knowledge base and developing a sense of mastery over how all of these factors—insulin, food, exercise, etc.—affect your blood glucose level can take years of experience. Remember that despite advances in diabetes treatment, we still rely on imperfect tools to manage type 1 diabetes. There is no magic formula for getting perfect blood glucose numbers, and no one with diabetes can have a blood glucose level constantly between 80 and 120 mg/dl. Be kind to yourself and avoid yearning for perfection. Setting goals that are out of reach is the road to frustration. There will be some periods in life, such as during pregnancy, when you will be highly motivated and your priority will be ensuring excellent glucose control, but these are temporary situations that prove impossible to sustain over a lifetime.

Having realistic goals is the key to living well in all aspects of life, and your diabetes self-care is no different. If your personal blood glucose goal is to stay between 70 and 180 mg/dl, aim for the *average* of your blood glucose measurements to be in that range. This does not necessarily mean that all, or even most, of your individual measurements will fall into that target range. Instead, the information you gain from frequent blood glucose monitoring will give you tips on how to approach your treatment regimen. It helps you spot trends in your glucose levels, so you can optimize your treatment. It's so you can determine how much insulin you need in a given dose, whether you're safe to drive a car, or whether you need to eat more snacks to treat hypoglycemia. Regardless, remember that blood glucose monitoring is not a test of whether you are a "good" or "bad" patient. Many people think this, but nothing could be further from the truth. Your blood glucose levels provide some insight into what needs to be done to improve your diabetes self-care, not to suggest that you're a bad person or that you've failed in taking care of yourself.

However, just because no one can achieve perfect numbers does not mean that you should give up on doing your best. You do have control over many aspects of your diabetes care, and the things you do control can make a huge difference in how you feel today and in your future health. It's important to become confident that you have control over your glucose levels. At the same time, remember that our bodies do not always respond as anticipated, no matter what you do. Even individuals who have lived with diabetes for decades can have the rug pulled out from under them by mysterious and unexplainable blood glucose fluctuations. When this happens, you will likely become frustrated. This is exactly when you need to go easy on yourself. Take a deep breath, wait awhile, and start over from the beginning.

Hypoglycemia

Whenever there is more insulin circulating than the body needs, there is a risk that your blood glucose level will go low. The result is a low blood glucose reaction called hypoglycemia. Sometimes it can be difficult figuring out how much insulin to take, and therefore, hypoglycemic episodes are an inevitable side effect of insulin use. The risk for hypoglycemia increases when one strives to keep average blood glucose levels close to the normal range. The common symptoms of hypoglycemia include perspiration, jitteriness, and rapid heartbeats, but there are countless others. Sometimes, if blood glucose levels dip low enough, brain function becomes impaired, which can affect a person's ability to safely perform common activities, such as driving a car. Moreover, hypoglycemia can have other dangerous effects, such as seizures, coma, and even death. One dangerous side effect of having frequent hypoglycemic episodes is that it becomes more difficult to detect hypoglycemia, a condition known as *hypoglycemia unawareness.* Hypoglycemia unawareness presents a particularly risky situation for people with diabetes because their blood glucose levels can go dangerously low before the situation is recognized and treated.

SOME COMMON CAUSES OF HYPOGLYCEMIA

- Too much mealtime insulin in relation to the amount of carbohydrate eaten.
- Exercise without sufficient snacking or sufficient reduction in the insulin dose.
- Alcohol use.
- Erratic absorption of insulin. This is particularly a problem with the long-acting insulins, such as NPH, and is often the underlying cause of reactions that occur overnight.
- Taking excessive amounts of insulin to bring down elevated blood glucose levels.
- Slow emptying of the stomach.

STEPS TO REDUCE THE TOLL OF HYPOGLYCEMIA

- Join a diabetes self-management education program to better understand how insulin acts in the body and how to match your insulin dose with food and exercise. Getting involved in such an education program is often the key to success for many individuals with frequent episodes of hypoglycemia. However, even with a good mastery of all of these factors, avoiding hypoglycemia can be a frustratingly difficult task.

- Wear a Medic-Alert chain or bracelet so that if you are ever unable to ask for help, the people who might help you (such as paramedics) will know that you have diabetes and will be able to give you appropriate care.

- Change to an insulin program that gives more predictable insulin absorption, such as an insulin pump or basal-bolus injection therapy with Lantus. There is evidence that frequent hypoglycemia leads to hypoglycemia unawareness and that by minimizing the frequency of your hypoglycemic reactions you can get your warning symptoms back.

- Enroll in hypoglycemia awareness training.

- Ensure that your friends and significant others know about the treatment of hypoglycemia, including use of glucagon.

- Help your family and friends understand that you do not have 100% control over hypoglycemic episodes. If they think it is entirely under your control, their worry and concern for your health and safety might be expressed as "blame and shame" (some examples: "Why do you keep doing this to yourself?", "Don't you care about yourself?", "Don't you know how ridiculous you act when you're low?", "Do you want to keep embarrassing me?"). It is also critical that a spouse or roommate who feels frightened by the idea of hypoglycemia have the opportunity to discuss this with your health care providers. This can help prevent blood glucose levels or hypoglycemia from becoming a source of tension in your relationships with others.

Weight and Blood Glucose

When your average blood glucose levels come down, there is a possibility of weight gain. However, it's also important to keep in mind that many strategies can make it much easier to control your weight (through diet and exercise) without sacrificing blood glucose control. Let's review how intensive insulin therapy can lead to weight gain.

- *High average blood glucose levels require more calories to be consumed.* When the glucose level goes over 180 mg/dl, some excess glucose will spill over into the urine. Consequently, some of the calories taken in are lost and not used for energy. As a result, individuals with suboptimally controlled diabetes generally tend to eat more calories than the body needs.

- *Blood glucose levels in the target range require fewer calories to provide the same amount of energy.* Once glucose levels get back into your target range (the goal of intensive therapy), fewer calories are lost in the urine. Therefore, if you continue to eat as much as you did when your blood glucose levels were not as carefully controlled, these extra calories will start adding up and lead to weight gain. In addition, there is evidence that when glucose levels are in the target range, your body uses calories more efficiently. As a result, fewer calories are needed to provide energy for the body. In short, in optimizing your blood glucose levels, you will also need to modify your diet.

▪ *Treating hypoglycemia requires snacks, and snacks mean more calories.* With tight glucose control comes the increased risk for hypoglycemia. The snacks taken to treat these reactions means added calories (especially if you eat until you feel better rather than following the 15-15 rule, in which you take 15 grams of carbohydrate, wait 15 minutes, and check your blood glucose level to see if you should repeat treatment).

In many ways, it may seem that in treating your diabetes, you're caught in a terrible catch-22 involving weight gain and working to optimize your blood glucose levels. This process does take work, and the risk of weight gain is present, but you need to remember that you can prevent weight gain. Changing to a basal-bolus insulin program (either with injections or the pump) can help you keep off extra pounds. Here's how:

▪ If the Lantus dose and pump basal rates are set correctly, there should be no need for snacks between meals.

▪ With a basal-bolus program, you can more precisely control the amount of insulin taken at mealtime, making it easier to go on a diet.

■ Also, the more precise control of insulin levels with a basal-bolus program makes it easier to avoid hypoglycemia, which means fewer snacks (and unwanted calories) to treat hypoglycemic episodes.

■ Insulin pump therapy offers an extra advantage when it comes to weight control. With a pump, you can reduce the basal rates during activity, especially during exercise. This means that you won't need to snack as often to cover the glucose expended during exercise; therefore, individuals using the pump can burn off unwanted calories more effectively through exercise.

Keep in mind that what you eat really does count. In the past, before basal-bolus insulin therapy and carbohydrate counting, the rules were "no sugar, no candy, and no doughnuts unless you're low." That old rule has changed. Carbohydrate counting now offers enough flexibility to give you the freedom to eat just about whatever you want. Unfortunately, this leads many people to incorrectly assume that they can eat whatever they want, whenever, and in whatever amount as long as the food is covered by extra insulin. This type of thinking can lead straight to weight gain. Even when using carbohydrate counting, people with diabetes need to watch what they eat.

As you work toward improving your diabetes control and mastering carbohydrate counting, try not to lose sight of the healthy eating goals for which all people should strive. It's easy to get so caught up in carbohydrate counting and bolus calculations that you forget that you also need to focus on good nutrition and other factors, such as the fat content and calories in your food. Remember, fats pack in over twice as many calories as protein or carbohydrates, so restricting your fat intake can also help in keeping the lid on your overall calorie intake.

Many adolescents with diabetes experience weight gain as insulin doses are increased during the years of puberty. This may have happened to you, too. Weight gain from this period may have left you with an understandable fear of taking insulin. However, you now have no reason to hold onto this fear because during puberty your body was naturally less responsive (more resistant) to insulin and you required higher doses. That period of your life is over now, and your young-adult body will be more responsive to insulin. Unfortunately, many teens do not have their insulin dose reduced after puberty. Thus, their insulin dose is much higher than they need, and they develop the habit of "eating up" to their insulin dose. In the past, you may have felt that you had to sacrifice blood glucose control to maintain your weight. Feeling that way is counterproductive to optimizing blood glucose control, and your health care team should take measures to ensure that your insulin doses meet your insulin needs.

During puberty, you may have also felt that no matter how hard you tried, you could not control your blood glucose. Keeping your blood glucose levels in a consistent range is always a demanding task, but it is especially difficult during puberty because the body is less sensitive to insulin. Young adults with these worries are more likely to struggle with eating and weight control. If you feel that you are struggling with these issues, please let your diabetes team know. You are certainly not alone, and there are lots of ways to help you out of this vicious cycle.

This is why it is so important to meet with a nutritionist or registered dietitian now that you are a young adult. Doing so will ensure that your daily calorie intake is appropriate for your current insulin needs. Also, you may feel very uncomfortable discussing your weight with your health care team, but you should try as hard as you can to make this discussion happen. Whether you are male or female, it is very important that your diabetes team understands how you feel about your weight and your shape. As a first step, speak with a nutritionist about your weight concerns. Then, let all of your providers know that you want to focus on the twin goals of optimal weight *and* optimal blood glucose control. Your health care team is there to help you in many of your needs. Combining the knowledge and skills of your multidisciplinary diabetes team with your personal goals and experience makes reaching an optimal weight and optimizing your blood glucose a very realistic goal.

For more pointers on healthy eating, check this out:
The College Student's Guide to Eating Well on Campus,
by Ann Selkowitz Litt, Tulip Hill Press, 2005.

COMPLICATIONS AND PREVENTION

There's a good chance that you've heard more about diabetes complications than you'd care to know. So many stories about diabetes complications circulate that it can be difficult to tell which ones are true. Here are some of the most important things to know when it comes to diabetes complications.

- Yes, it's true that diabetes is the most common cause for blindness in the industrialized world.

- Yes, it's true that people with diabetes are 20 times more likely to have kidney failure than people without diabetes.

- Yes, it's true that individuals with diabetes are more likely to have limb and foot problems related to neuropathy (nerve damage) and poor circulation.

On the other hand, doom and gloom do not surround everything concerning diabetes. Keep these facts in mind, too.

- Most of the information we have about diabetes complications comes from groups of patients who did not have access to blood glucose monitoring or intensive diabetes treatment regimens early in their course of living with diabetes.

- Complications *are not* inevitable.

- Complications *can* be prevented and sometimes reversed.

- Complications *do not* develop overnight. In fact, complications take years to develop, so occasional lapses in your diabetes control are not going to instantly give you complications.

- *Any* improvement in diabetes control can help reduce the risk for complications.

Retinopathy (Eye Disease)

Retinopathy—damage to the retina, the light-sensing part of the inner eye—is one of the more common complications of diabetes. The Diabetes Control and Complications Trial (DCCT) conclusively showed that glucose control is an important factor in the development of retinopathy. For every 1% reduction in A1C (a test that provides an average blood glucose level over a 2- to 3-month period), there was a 40% reduction in the risk for retinopathy. This should illustrate that every improvement in your blood glucose control counts. You don't have to achieve an A1C of 6.8% to benefit from a lower risk of retinopathy; just lowering your A1C from 9.5% to 8.5% will give you a big dividend.

It should also be noted that although high glucose levels contribute to the development of eye disease, not all individuals with suboptimal diabetes control necessarily develop eye disease. Some 43% of the individuals in the DCCT with A1C levels over 9.5% did not have eye disease. In fact, only 1.8% of the patients with A1C levels over 9.5% did develop the more severe signs of retinopathy. This tells us that high blood glucose levels contribute to the development of eye disease, but that other factors (such as high blood pressure and your genes) also play a role.

Too often, individuals who get complications end up blaming themselves (and their loved ones may blame them as well). This can turn into a vicious downward spiral in which you blame yourself for something you may not have been able to control and can lead to feelings of depression. Depression can be problematic for people with diabetes because when people often feel depressed, they have

Figure 4: Effect of A1C on the Development of Retinopathy (Diabetic Eye Disease)

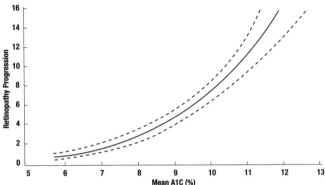

less energy and less interest in caring for themselves. This can lead to devoting less time and attention to diabetes self-care. It is important to try and prevent this cycle from developing. Keep in mind that if only some people with high A1C values develop severe retinopathy, then it makes more sense to blame your genes than it does to blame yourself and your blood glucose. In addition, if you do develop retinopathy, the most important thing you can do to prevent this complication from becoming worse is to continue to check your blood glucose levels, continue to take your insulin, and continue to see your diabetes team.

Remember that having some eye damage (retinopathy) from diabetes does not mean that you are going to become blind. With the tools available today, such as laser therapy and vitrectomy surgery, the risk for distinct visual loss has been substantially reduced. To illustrate this, one recent report studied about 600 individuals with type 1 diabetes who were diagnosed between 1965 and 1984 and were followed over a 20-year period. Only seven individuals in this group became blind from retinopathy. Moreover, the 244 individuals diagnosed with type 1 diabetes between 1979 and 1984 had an average A1C of 8.5%. Despite this less-than-perfect glucose control, by the end of the follow-up period, *none* of these individuals developed blindness from retinopathy. All of these individuals had their blood pressure carefully monitored and had their eyes examined at least every year by an ophthalmologist (eye specialist). There is evidence that blood pressure control can have an important impact in preserving vision. In the United Kingdom Prospective Diabetes Study (a trial in individuals with type 2 diabetes), it was found that tight blood pressure control was associated with a 47% reduced risk for deterioration of vision. In short, this means that your blood glucose levels, while very important, do not directly reflect any chance that you'll go blind from retinopathy. In fact, blood pressure control may be more important in controlling retinopathy than blood glucose levels. Does this mean you can ignore your blood glucose levels? Certainly not! Plenty of studies have shown that you are still at an increased risk of developing retinopathy if you do not control your blood glucose levels.

It is important to know that you won't notice any change in your vision when retinopathy first develops, so it's critical that you get your eyes examined at least annually. Early detection of retinopathy leads to early treatment, which can preserve vision.

PREVENTING VISUAL LOSS FROM DIABETES

- ◼ If you have had type 1 diabetes for more than 3 years, have a dilated eye exam at least annually.

- ◼ If you do have retinopathy, check with your health care provider to make sure that your blood pressure is well controlled.

- ◼ Strive for the best glucose control you can achieve.

Nephropathy (Kidney Disease)

The final stages of nephropathy (kidney damage caused by diabetes) result in kidney failure and can only be treated in one of two ways: dialysis or a kidney transplant. For this reason, people with diabetes tend to fear this potentially fatal complication the most. Be assured, however, that nephropathy takes years to develop, so kidney failure does not spring up suddenly without advance warning. During the earliest phase of nephropathy, the damaged kidneys start leaking small amounts of a protein called albumin into the urine. This is referred to as microalbuminuria. At this early stage, the kidneys are still functioning normally. Although microalbuminuria is an early sign of changes in the kidneys, microalbuminuria *does not* necessarily lead to kidney failure. Several studies have shown that individuals with microalbuminuria who take a drug known as an angiotensin-converting enzyme (ACE) inhibitor (a blood pressure medication) can prevent diabetes from causing further damage and prevent any deterioration in kidney function. In fact, recent studies indicate that microalbuminuria can go away if properly treated. Use of ACE inhibitors, careful control of blood pressure, and improved glucose control (A1C less than 8%) are the key factors associated with improved kidney function.

Like retinopathy, the development of nephropathy usually goes unnoticed, so it's critical that you get your urine checked for microalbumin at least annually. Early detection leads to early treatment, and this can prevent kidney failure.

PREVENTING KIDNEY DAMAGE FROM DIABETES

- Be sure that your urine is checked for microalbumin every year.
- If microalbuminuria is confirmed on repeated testing of the urine, be sure that you start taking an ACE inhibitor drug.
- Be sure to check with your health care provider that your blood pressure is well controlled.
- Strive for the best glucose control you can achieve.

DON'T JUMP TO CONCLUSIONS

The urine microalbumin test can pick up the earliest signs of damage to the kidneys. This test allows for very early treatment of kidney disease, meaning that you can begin ACE inhibitor treatment before there is any permanent change in kidney function. Unfortunately, the urine microalbumin test can sometimes be mistakenly positive. False-positive results can occur when you have been active (simply rushing into your appoint-

continued on page 36

continued from page 35

ment can cause this), you have high blood glucose, or you have a fever or urinary tract infection. For women, menstruation can induce false-positive results on the test. For these reasons, do not panic if your urine microalbumin test shows elevated levels of protein in the urine. Instead, ensure that a repeat test confirms the results before you receive treatment for the early signs of nephropathy.

Feet

You have probably heard the statistics surrounding the increased risks for foot ulcers and amputations associated with diabetes. However, few people are told that most severe foot problems associated with diabetes are *preventable* and usually arise because they seek treatment too late. Normally, foot ulcers and amputations begin with untreated wounds or injuries to the foot, which go unnoticed because of loss of feeling in the limbs. With some relatively simple measures, it is possible for you to ensure that you never become part of these statistics. Clinical examinations performed every 3 months can help you learn more about your risk for foot problems.

- If your physician can find a good, healthy pulse (your heart beat) in different parts of your feet (showing that you have good circulation) and you can feel a 10-gram monofilament (a small flexible fiber used to test nerve sensitivity), then you have a low risk of developing foot problems.

- If you can't feel the monofilament, then there is a risk that you may injure yourself and not feel any pain. This can turn into a problem if damage to your skin or foot goes unnoticed and untreated—sometimes resulting in an ulcer, infection, or foot deformity. In addition, if the pulses in your foot are reduced, this indicates that blood flow to the feet is impaired and healing is likely to be slowed.

PREVENTING FOOT PROBLEMS FROM DIABETES

- Don't go barefoot, and inspect your feet daily, especially between the toes. These are good habits for everyone with diabetes, but particularly for those who have lost some sensation and don't feel the monofilament very well.

- Make a habit of cutting your toenails straight across. This helps prevent ingrown toenails.

- If you notice any foot problems (such as redness, an open sore, or a puncture wound) call your doctor immediately. As with all possible complications, early treatment prevents them from developing into a serious problem.

- If you smoke, quit. Cigarette smoking is a major cause for circulatory problems in individuals who have diabetes.

Summary

The best investments you can make to avoid diabetes complications are to *1)* work with your diabetes team to improve your blood glucose control and *2)* continue to see your diabetes team and receive diabetes health care (including annual check-ups). Doing this throughout the young-adult years allows you to take advantage of new treatments for the early signs of complications. Frequent examinations also increase the chances that the early signs of any complication will be discovered, ensuring timely preventive treatment.

SOME ADVICE FOR YOUR JOURNEY

You now know what tasks await you as you pass into your young-adult years, but here's some advice to make achieving them easier.

▨ *It will take some time for all of your diabetes self-care tasks to become an automatic part of your daily routine.* Achieving good diabetes care will always demand extra effort, which adds even more tasks to your already-busy schedule. With this many duties to attend to, it's easy to get burned out by these new demands and then decide that the effort isn't worthwhile. Don't let this happen to you. Remember that mastering the new tools of diabetes management is like learning to drive a car. Initially, every action will be conscious, deliberate, and probably stressful. However, after some time, you'll become confident in managing your diabetes, and these extra tasks will become an automatic (and almost unconscious) part of your daily routine. Avoid diabetes burnout by setting realistic goals and remaining patient.

▨ *Don't view lapses as a sign of failure.* For most people with diabetes, the road to improved care is not direct or smooth. In short, optimizing your blood glucose will not be easy or immediate, so give yourself some latitude. There will be times when other demands take a greater priority in your life than diabetes (such as final exams, starting a new job, or moving away from home). On these occasions, one's focus on diabetes tends to lapse, and blood glucose control suffers. This is acceptable if your blood glucose levels don't fluctuate too greatly and as long as you get back on track when the stressful period ends. Be sure that you guard against letting these lapses lead to a total relapse, in which you lose confidence in your ability to manage your blood glucose and give up. People who give up begin skipping the regular duties of diabetes self-care, such as blood glucose monitoring, injections, and appointments, and avoid their diabetes team. This presents a dangerous situation for the person with diabetes.

Many people (and not just those with diabetes) misunderstand diabetes self-care, seeing it as a series of black-and-white decisions. Where else in your life is it a failure if you do something and then decide that it was not really the best choice? Aren't those what we call learning experiences? Don't they help us make better choices in the future? Thinking of your diabetes self-care as a simple pass-fail test will not lead to success. Like all things in life, you need to approach your self-care as a lifelong learning process, one in which you'll get better, but probably after you've made a few mistakes.

You may experience a single, brilliant moment when you realize the importance of getting on track, but learning how to manage your diabetes does not happen quite as quickly, not overnight or even in six months. Mastering this process takes time. There will be times when you fall back into your old patterns of diabetes management. Don't beat yourself up; it's normal and human to do this. Don't punish yourself for being human. Instead, recognize that these old methods were not particularly useful and that the newer ways are more likely to help you achieve your goals.

■ *Set attainable goals.* Mastering the intricacies of diabetes management (i.e., balancing insulin doses, food, and physical activity) takes time and effort. Even if your ultimate goal is to get your A1C down to 7.0%, it's important that you start by working with your diabetes team to set an attainable goal. As you succeed in your efforts, you'll become more confident in your skills and feel encouraged to further advance your goals. For example, if you currently have an A1C of 9.0%, then it may be better to start off with a goal A1C of 8.0% and later aim for 7.0%. Guard against giving yourself unrealistic goals. When you set your sights on something unattainable, failure and frustration will likely be the only results. Sometimes, this leads to the conclusion that the effort isn't even worthwhile, which is the worst possible decision if you are trying to improve your diabetes care. This is why reasonable, sensible, and attainable goals will be the key to success in life and in your diabetes self-care. After all, did you begin college expecting to finish in 3 years and to make the Dean's List every semester? You probably knew that this was not a realistic goal. Realistically, you should strive to do your best, discover an area that interests you, and balance your school work with a social life. Attainable goals also allow you to reach your goals safely, an important factor in making changes to your health. Also, remember that it's best to set your primary goals around new behavior patterns (or habits) rather than a new blood glucose goal. Your blood glucose levels will improve if you focus on frequent blood glucose monitoring, so make that your goal. If you just plan to lower your A1C level to 8.0%, but don't think about how you'll do it, you're setting yourself up for frustration.

■ *Everyone adjusts to new diabetes behaviors at a different pace.* No doubt, your pace in achieving your diabetes self-care goals will be different from other people's paces. This shouldn't be surprising. For you to determine how quickly to move toward your goals, start by identifying the demands on your life that you must meet and the external barriers you face (such as work duties or "crush time" in classes). You should also look at your own internal barriers (e.g., worrying about hypoglycemia, worrying about weight), which you will have to confront. It is important to discuss these demands and barriers with your diabetes team as you work together to set realistic and achievable diabetes-specific goals. Your health care team may ask you to fill out the PAID (Problem Areas in Diabetes; see box on this page) questionnaire to help you identify some of these hurdles. Obviously, you should try to get your diabetes care on track sooner rather than later, but effecting change also takes time. So be patient!

POTHOLES AND SPEED BUMPS ON THE ROAD OF LIVING WITH DIABETES

The following list contains items from the PAID questionnaire, listed in order of most worrisome to least worrisome in a sample population of

continued on page 42

continued from page 41

adults with diabetes. Read through these items and look to see where these items rate in your life. Doing so will help you get a head start in developing realistic goals.

1. Worrying about the future and the possibility of serious complications.
2. Feeling guilty or anxious when you get off track with your diabetes management.
3. Feeling scared when you think about living with diabetes.
4. Feeling discouraged with your diabetes regimen.
5. Worrying about low blood glucose reactions.
6. Feeling constantly burned out by the constant effort to manage diabetes.
7. Not knowing if the mood or feelings you are experiencing are related to your blood glucose.
8. Coping with complications of diabetes.
9. Feeling constantly concerned about food.
10. Feeling depressed when you think about living with diabetes.
11. Feeling angry when you think about living with diabetes.
12. Feeling overwhelmed by your diabetes regimen.
13. Feeling alone with diabetes.
14. Feelings of deprivation regarding food and meals.

15. Not having clear and concrete goals for your diabetes care.

16. Uncomfortable interactions about diabetes with family and/or friends.

17. Not accepting diabetes.

18. Feeling that friends and/or family are not supportive of diabetes management efforts.

19. Feeling unsatisfied with your diabetes physician.

PREPARING FOR THE COLLEGE YEARS

When you leave home for college, be prepared to take care of yourself. Using the following tips will give you the information and preparation you need to be ready for most situations.

Before you head off to school, pack a *Campus Diabetes Kit*. It should contain the following:

- Glucose monitor and strips.

- Insulin vials.

- Syringes or pump supplies (such as reservoirs, insertion sets).

- Sharps container.

- A ready source of glucose to treat hypoglycemia, such as juice, glucose tablets, or glucose gel. Remember, vending machines aren't always around and aren't always reliable.

continued on page 44

continued from page 43

- Medical identification (such as a Medic-Alert ID bracelet)—this may not be your first pick as a fashion statement, but if you're ever unconscious, it may be your lifeline.

- Important contact numbers (take a supply of business cards from your current diabetes care team to share with your new health care providers and emergency room staff).

- Prescriptions for diabetes supplies.

As you get settled into school, here are some key things to do.

- Decide who to tell and what to tell about your diabetes. The next section, "Young Adult Relationships and Diabetes," will provide more information on this subject.

- Meet with the student health service and find out how to access night, weekend, and emergency services.

- Find the cafeteria and other eating places. Obtain the nutrition information for the available foods. It may be worthwhile to set up your own dorm room food supply, just in case the food available doesn't meet your health needs.

- Prepare a "Dorm Room Sick-Day Kit." It should include your sick-day guidelines for adjusting insulin, ketone strips, a thermometer, and a nutrition stock consisting of bland foods and liquids (such as juice, sugar-free beverages, crackers, and broth-based soups).

YOUNG-ADULT RELATIONSHIPS AND DIABETES

In the past, your parents likely spoke for you and your diabetes. They probably did this with everyone, including your teachers, family, friends, and health care team. Now, as a young adult, you are the one who needs to talk about diabetes. You need to make the three vital decisions in letting others know about diabetes: *1)* who to tell, *2)* what to tell, and *3)* when to tell.

1. *Who to tell?* In some cases, disclosing your diabetes is a legal requirement, such as when you fill out insurance forms, driver's license applications, and college or employment health inventories. However, in most social situations, disclosing your diabetes is an option. You need to develop a plan covering *who to tell*. As a general rule, it is most important to discuss your diabetes with the people with whom you spend a lot of time (such as roommates, close friends, lab partners, sports coaches, and teammates). It is important that they understand that you have insulin-dependent diabetes and that you work hard to take care of your blood glucose, but sometimes you may have a hypoglycemic episode in which you may seem different, confused, or even out of it. Let them know how to help you with a sudden low blood glucose episode by telling them where you keep your supplies and meter and who they should contact in an emergency. This information safety net will let you go about the business of being an active young adult.

2. *What to tell?* You will need to have a plan about what or how much you should tell other people about diabetes. A lot of times,

your personal comfort level with these people will determine this. In other cases, such as with employers, coaches, and teachers, it is in your best interest to tell them enough to allow them to treat you in an emergency.

Some people with diabetes find it helpful to ask someone if they have ever known anyone with type 1 diabetes. Another helpful question is to ask what that person knows about diabetes, particularly type 1 diabetes. This gives you a chance to hear their beliefs, their information, and possibly their misinformation about diabetes. With this knowledge, you can then respond to their personal experiences and knowledge and add in the important bits of information that you feel are important. For example, this may be the moment to tell them that you wear an insulin pump to provide continuous insulin to the body or that you often check your blood glucose so you can avoid high and low blood glucose.

3. *When to tell?* Again, it is your decision when to tell someone about your diabetes. There is, of course a spectrum of times when you may want to bring up your diabetes, just like there are different times when you may wish to bring up other personal information. (For example, if your parents are divorced, then you probably don't mention this in your first conversation with someone.) However, as a rule of thumb, if you find you are spending lots of energy keeping your diabetes a secret and feel lots of tension in trying to hide your diabetes tasks in social situations or within relationships, then it may be time to talk openly about your diabetes. You will develop your own timing style as your social circle expands to include new acquaintances, friends, and co-

workers. Your confidence will grow as you receive responses that let you know you made the right decision.

Changing Ties with Your Family

Your family ties—with your siblings, aunts and uncles, grandparents, and, most noticeably, parents—will change as you move through the young-adult period. For any young adult, this can be a confusing time as you try to figure out just how your family fits into your life as an adult. Having diabetes adds another entire level to these changing relationships. In particular, it is important that you continue to have appropriate support from your family. Here are some lessons from other young adults and their families that may help you.

- Keep your parents informed about your new diabetes care provider. Keep them informed about your overall health. Doing this will relieve some of their worry and may help keep them off of your back. When you let your parents know that you are working with a health care team, they can see that you are working to take care of yourself.
- Diabetes management and care can be expensive. Learn to talk realistically about the financial help you will need to take the best care of your diabetes. You may not want to ask your family for help with the other expenses of daily living, but do not feel too proud to ask for help with the expenses of diabetes care.
- Talk with your parents and siblings about the aspects of your new life, and include diabetes as you speak about your roommate,

classes, work schedule, etc. Doing this lets your family know that you are integrating diabetes into your new life. Again, the less your family worries about your diabetes, the less nagging you'll receive from them. Honest and open communication will resolve many worries before they become problems.

- If necessary, you can keep your parents up to date on advances in diabetes treatment and research by referring them to articles, websites, and so forth. This indicates that you are continuing to learn about diabetes.

- If you are living at home, negotiate for the level of privacy that you feel you need. Ask for the support you need, too. This is not only important in regard to your diabetes-specific tasks, but to all areas of your life.

BUILDING AN EFFECTIVE RELATIONSHIP WITH YOUR ADULT-CARE PROVIDER

Moving on to a new health care provider involves more than just going to see a new doctor and leaving your parents behind. You may have strong attachments to your pediatrician that were forged over years and find that adult doctors can seem much colder and direct. Becoming accustomed to this new adult relationship may take some time. Making this relationship effective can take more time and some work.

Keep in mind that the relationships people with diabetes have with their health care providers differ greatly from the relationships found in people with other conditions. If you break your leg, for example, your doctor makes most of the decisions about what needs to be done to set the bones correctly. In contrast, when it comes to managing diabetes, you make the day-to-day decisions, and your health care provider takes on the role of a coach, giving you tips on how to perform better. Ultimately, you decide whether you will follow his or her advice.

Clearly, this is a two-way street. On the one hand, you will have to accept much more responsibility for your self-care—no one will remind you to check your blood glucose or make sure you make it to your check-ups. Conversely, your provider needs to understand that his or her role is to guide you in your decisions rather than tell you what to do. You should expect your health care provider to coach you and refrain from being judgmental. At the same time, your health care provider should be able to expect that you will take on more responsibility in caring for yourself.

For your part, a helpful habit is to begin writing a checklist for your visits to your health care provider. Your checklist should include:

- *Practical matters.* Write down things you need or need to know for daily life. This includes prescriptions, advice about that new glucose monitor you read about, the travel letter you'll need for your upcoming vacation, and so forth.

- *Diabetes matters.* Write down issues that concern diabetes itself and self-management. What has been on your mind about diabetes? What issues have come up since your last visit to your provider? Maybe you've decided you want to tighten up on your diabetes control and you want to discuss where to begin. Maybe you are concerned about how hypoglycemic reactions could affect your relationship with your significant other—ask him or her to accompany you to your next visit. Or maybe you have concerns about your weight and want to discuss healthy weight-loss strategies.

■ *Prevention.* Write down important dates so you don't forget them, such as when to schedule annual exams (e.g., dilated eye test, urine test, and A1C test). Also write down signs and symptoms that are new or different, which may suggest complications. As you already know, the complications of diabetes can be prevented and reversed. The key is early detection.

HEALTH INSURANCE ISSUES

It is inevitable that you will have to deal with your health insurance company. Try not to be overwhelmed by the complex processes of health insurance, and seek help whenever you feel you don't understand what's going on with your insurance. The ins and outs of insurance can take a while to understand, so here are some tips to help you.

■ Some managed care plans won't cover nonemergency expenses out of the plan's geographic area. Therefore, if you're thinking of going to a school or just living away from home, it's important to find out if your health insurance will cover you in your new location.

- Some college-sponsored health plans do not cover *preexisting conditions* (such as diabetes) or the cost of outpatient prescription drugs. Before enrolling, it's important to find out if this will affect you.

- Many plans will allow young adults to remain on their parents' health insurance policy up until the age of 25 years, provided they are full-time students (which must be verified by the school) and remain unmarried.

Here are two helpful websites:

- http://www.slba.com
  The website for Stephen L. Beckley and Associates, Inc., has a nice page full of information on choosing college student health insurance.

- http://www.acha.org/info_resources/stu_health_ins.pdf
  This page from the American College Health Association provides their standards for student health insurance and benefits.

OTHER ISSUES TO THINK ABOUT

Pregnancy Requires Preparation

Remarkable advances in technology have made having a healthy pregnancy and healthy newborn a tangible reality for young women with diabetes. However, excessively high blood glucose levels can cause newborn babies to have birth defects, so very careful blood glucose control is a necessity. Women should strive for the lowest

A1C level possible (without causing hypoglycemia) when they are trying to get pregnant. If you are going to try to become pregnant, meet with your health care team beforehand to discuss what steps must be taken to ensure a safe and healthy pregnancy.

This should underscore the value of effective contraception. An unintended pregnancy may result in birth defects (because you haven't been preparing by optimizing your blood glucose), so choose birth control carefully. Note that there are no contraceptive methods that are specifically off-limits to women with diabetes, but effectiveness should be a priority.

"WHAT'S THE CHANCE THAT MY CHILDREN WILL HAVE DIABETES?"

Many individuals with type 1 diabetes ask this question and do so for understandable reasons. Unfortunately, no clear-cut answer truly exists. The data vary slightly from one study to another. Research performed at the Joslin Clinic indicates that if the father has type 1 diabetes, then there's about a 5% risk that his children will develop type 1 diabetes. On the other hand, if the mother has type 1 diabetes, then this risk is only about 2%.

The risk also appears to vary depending on the age of the parent when he or she was diagnosed with diabetes. For example, if the father was diagnosed with diabetes before age 11 years, the risk is 9%. Conversely, if the father was diagnosed after 11 years of age, the risk is 4%. Mothers show different risks in different ages as well. If a mother is diagnosed with diabetes before age 11 years, the risk is 3%. If diagnosis comes after age 11 years, the risk is 2%. Interestingly, data also show that a mother's age at pregnancy provides additional concern. For women with type 1 diabetes aged 25 years or more at the time of the pregnancy, the likelihood that their children will develop type 1 diabetes drops to less than 1%, a level of risk almost as low as that for people without diabetes. Therefore, young women with type 1 diabetes may greatly benefit from waiting to have children, and effective contraceptive use is very important to prevent unplanned pregnancies.

Smoking

Cigarette smoking becomes a temptation in the lives of too many adolescents and young adults, and those with diabetes are no different. Rather than give you a sermon on the perils of smoking, we'll give you the sobering facts. Smoking accounts for over 400,000 deaths in the U.S. per year and is the leading avoidable cause of death in this country. In individuals with diabetes, the added risks of smoking are even greater. For smokers with diabetes, the risk for developing nephropathy (kidney disease) from diabetes increases exponentially. Smoking greatly affects the circulatory system, which involves the heart and blood vessels. Thus, smoking adds to the risk for coronary artery disease (the major cause of death in people with diabetes) and can cause vascular and foot problems. It takes a while for smoking to cause irreversible damage, so it's never too late to quit.

Alcohol

Alcohol will likely be part of the social scene you encounter at college, so you need to understand how it can affect you and your diabetes. Binge drinking is not just something to dismiss as a passing phase. The consequences—hangovers, blackouts, losing control, and giving in to unplanned and unprotected sex—can be serious, whether or not you have diabetes. There is also evidence that excessive drinking can destroy brain function. Drinking and diabetes together can be an even more dangerous, and sometimes lethal, combination.

The impaired judgment that comes from even slight alcohol intoxication can cause you to make the wrong decisions about managing your diabetes. So, even a slight buzz isn't anything to just shrug off. In addition, alcohol can directly affect glucose metabolism in your body. Alcoholic beverages can cause hypoglycemia and high blood glucose (hyperglycemia).

▪ *Alcohol can block the liver from releasing glucose, leading to hypoglycemia.* We previously mentioned that between meals and overnight the liver continuously releases glucose into your circulation. When the liver metabolizes alcohol (which can take hours for a single drink), glucose production is blocked. This results in hypoglycemia. So whenever you have alcohol, be prepared to snack—and make it a carbohydrate snack, like pretzels, rather than a high-fat snack, like cheese or peanuts—and cut back on your insulin dose. Remember, a single drink can have this effect. In addition, alcohol will block your liver from responding to glucagon, so if you go low from alcohol, your glucagon emergency kit won't be of much help.

◻ *Some alcoholic drinks contain a lot of carbohydrates and this can lead to hyperglycemia.* Beer, sweet wines, and mixed drinks made with fruit juices or regular soda can be full of carbohydrates. Such drinks may initially cause a rise in your blood glucose level, followed by a drop in blood glucose once the alcohol begins affecting the liver. Avoiding hypoglycemia is the priority if you drink. When you have carbohydrate-rich alcoholic drinks, do not take insulin to cover the carbohydrates.

SOME PRACTICAL TIPS FOR DRINKING

◻ Be realistic. You will probably enter social situations where drinking will be the norm, so plan ahead. Check with your health care provider ahead of time to find out what specific guidelines you should follow to adjust your insulin and snacking for these occasions.

◻ Always have food in your stomach when you drink alcohol. Food will slow down the absorption of alcohol into the bloodstream and reduce the amount that reaches the liver.

◻ Be prepared for hypoglycemia, not only while you drink, but also for hours afterward. Be sure to have carbohydrate snacks around when drinking. If possible, have a large snack before going to sleep after

continued on page 56

continued from page 55

you've been drinking. Monitor, monitor, and monitor more. Before going to sleep, set your alarm to wake you up a few hours later so you can check your blood glucose again. If you don't think you'll wake up to an alarm, ask your roommate or partner to check up on you.

■ Think twice before you have more than one drink. Alcohol and diabetes add up to more than double danger. Intoxication (drunkenness) leads to impaired judgment, and when your judgment is clouded, you may not notice the signs of hypoglycemia. As often happens, others may also attribute the signs of hypoglycemia to drunkenness, not realizing that you are in need of treatment. In most situations, you'll most likely have to rely on yourself to notice low blood glucose. This can be a dangerous situation, so be careful with alcohol.

3

For the Care Provider: Clinical Principles

GLYCEMIC CONTROL AND THE PATIENT-PROVIDER RELATIONSHIP

The conclusive evidence from several multicenter trials establishing a causal link between glycemic control and the microvascular complications of diabetes has highlighted the importance of the A1C level as a key predictor of future health. Inevitably, the focus of the interaction between clinician and patient has become increasingly directed around blood glucose monitoring records and A1C measurements. However, despite the evidence that metabolic control matters, tight glycemic control remains an elusive goal for many individual patients. Several studies have shown that diabetes self-management education without interventions to reinforce behavior change does not lead to sustained improvement in glycemic control. The median A1C of the intensive treatment cohort of the DCCT at 5 years after completion of the trial was 8.1% (up from 7.0–7.2% during the trial). Four years after the completion of the DCCT, the group of individuals who had been adolescents when enrolled into the intensive treatment limb of the study were young adults (aged 22–31 years) and had a mean A1C of 8.4%. These findings underscore the importance of considering the behavioral and developmental hurdles to maintaining tight glycemic control in the young-adult patient. Vinicor, who reviewed barriers to translation efforts, has emphasized that because patients with diabetes must take responsibility for their own care on a daily basis, successful approaches for implementing diabetes self-management must focus on promoting change in self-care behavior.

CLINICAL CHALLENGES OF YOUNG ADULTHOOD

For adolescents with tight glycemic control, the transition to young adulthood will often have only a minimal effect on the established routines of diabetes self-care. More often, however, adolescents will find that the growing responsibilities of young adulthood will distract from the demands of managing diabetes. Even when faced with the consequences of suboptimal glycemic control, some young adults will not be receptive to making major changes to their diabetes regimen. Reconciling this misfit between the demands of diabetes self-management and the developmental maturity of the young adult is a major challenge for the clinician.

Young-adult patients and their health care providers will often have different perceptions of the important priorities in care. Because the consequences of suboptimal glycemic control arise in the future, the asymptomatic young adult may not recognize the need for major changes in his or her diabetes regimen. Some young adults may feel that their new adult-care provider has unrealistic expectations and demands, and the fact that a bond of confidence and trust with this new physician has yet to be developed can heighten the young adult's concerns. The recommendations of the new physician may be interpreted as an intrusion into their autonomy and personal control, which can lead to estrangement from follow-up and care.

Realistic Expectations and Goals for the Clinician

- The clinical evaluation should include an assessment of the barriers to care (see "Uncover Barriers to Intensive Therapy" on page 67) and the competing demands of young-adult life. The treatment approach will need to be tailored to the young adult's expectations and receptiveness to change. (Is the patient just graduating to an adult provider? Is he or she expecting change? Is he or she even receptive to change?) This evaluation process can be aided by having the patient complete the Problem Areas in Diabetes (PAID) questionnaire beginning on page 41.

- The focus of care may need to be directed at ensuring continued medical follow-up, with annual urine microalbumin measurements and dilated eye examinations, and counseling for issues such as preparing for college, coping with the impact of diabetes on relationships, contraception, smoking, and alcohol use. Reviewing the "For the Young Adult" section will offer an overview of many of the subjects that might need to be covered in counseling sessions.

- Establishing a strong relationship based on acceptance and mutual respect can be critical in ensuring *1)* continued follow-up and *2)* the trust and influence that over time can promote improved self-care behavior. Retrospective studies have established that irregular clinic attendance and loss to medical follow-up are important predictors of the development of diabetic nephropathy. With maturation, the focus of the young adult gradually shifts toward making choices and plans for the future, and this will usually be accompanied by receptiveness to changing self-care behavior and improving glycemic control. This transition can be a rewarding window of opportunity for the clinician to shape the behavior that will determine the future health of the young patient. The early effort invested in developing a trusting relationship with the patient will often begin to reach fruition at this later stage.

A fundamental role of the health professional is to serve as the patient's guide in making informed choices about living with diabetes. This collaborative relationship between patient and provider should exist as a counterpart to the evolving relationship between parent and child during the transition from adolescence to young adulthood. An accepting and nonjudgmental approach by the clinician (i.e., respect for the patient's concerns and views and recognizing the burden and effort involved in living with diabetes) can set the foundation for a strong, lasting relationship. To emphasize that responsibility and control belong to the patient, it can be helpful to explicitly describe yourself as the patient's coach.

Adolescents and young adults are usually very sensitive to issues of control and personal autonomy. Threatening that growing individuality may isolate the patient, which is obviously counterproductive to care. If compliance with the provider's goals becomes the condition for approval and lapses in self-care and glycemic control are met with belittling or threatening comments, then the patient may become discouraged and disengage from care and medical follow-up.

EATING DISORDERS IN YOUNG ADULTS WITH DIABETES

A very important clinical challenge and barrier to care in young adults with diabetes is the possibility of developing eating disorders. Assessing possible eating disorders will require patience and a careful approach.

The Facts

- Although there is some controversy as to whether there is a greater prevalence of clinically diagnosable eating disorders (i.e., anorexia nervosa, bulimia nervosa, binge-eating disorder) among individuals with diabetes, recent research has shown that young women with diabetes have 2.4 times the risk of developing an eating disorder than age-matched women without diabetes. Several studies have also shown that about 30% of all women taking insulin struggle with subclinical symptoms of "disordered eating," such as restrictive eating, a preoccupation with weight and shape, feelings of guilt after eating, and strategic misuse of insulin for weight control.

- Clinically diagnosable eating disorders, such as anorexia, bulimia,

continued on page 62

continued from page 61

and subclinical disordered eating attitudes and behaviors, present a serious health risk to the patient with diabetes. Disordered eating is associated with poor metabolic control, problems in adherence, depression, increased risk of diabetic ketoacidosis (DKA), and increased rates of microvascular complications in women with diabetes.

■ Misuse of insulin for the purposes of weight control is such an effective weight-loss strategy that, once begun, it is almost impossible for young women to stop this high-risk behavior on their own.

■ Therefore, it is critical that diabetes clinicians understand the following:

1. How to prevent the development of disordered eating in their young-adult patients, especially females.
2. How to identify an eating disorder or disordered eating attitudes and behaviors.
3. How to work with a multidisciplinary team to intervene with the patient and family when a young-adult patient is struggling with an eating disorder or disordered eating.

Reducing the Risk of Disordered Eating

■ Negotiate realistic goals for blood glucose, weight, and behavior.

■ Avoid perfectionism.

■ Allow patients to express their negative feelings about having diabetes.

- Make it clear that it is normal to occasionally feel burdened or discouraged by the diabetes regimen.

- Refer to mental health providers if you suspect depression is causing or related to disordered eating.

- Listen to your patient's concerns about weight and shape.

- Be willing to work with your patients to help them reach realistic weight-loss goals.

- All members of the diabetes team should emphasize healthy eating, not dieting. The goal of a diabetes meal plan is flexibility, not restriction.

Identifying an Eating Disorder or Disordered Eating

Some early warning signs of eating disorders may include the following. (*Note*: These signs should raise your "index of suspicion" but are not definite signs of an eating disorder.)

- An unexplainable elevated A1C level in a patient knowledgeable about diabetes may indicate insulin misuse.

- Frequent DKA may be caused by insulin omission. Patients with serious eating disorders may learn how to avoid hospitalization for DKA by giving themselves only enough insulin to stay out of the hospital.

- Anxiety and avoidance concerning being weighed may indicate an eating disorder.

- Weight loss or weight maintenance when self-reported eating patterns should have caused weight gain.

continued on page 64

continued from page 63

■ Eating binges or alcohol abuse may occur alongside an eating disorder.

Because secrecy is a characteristic of most eating disorders, asking open-ended questions when one is suspected will help assess the possibility of a real disorder. Take the initiative with your patients and ask the following open-ended questions (adapted from Goebel-Fabbri, 2002).

■ "How do you feel about your body weight and shape?"

■ "How much do you currently weigh? How much would you like to weigh ideally? How often do you weigh yourself?"

■ "How do you like your current meal plan? Do you ever feel that it is too difficult to stick to this meal plan or that you are often eating too much or too little?"

■ "Do you ever change your insulin dose to influence your weight?"

■ "How many shots does your doctor recommend that you take each day, and how many shots do you take on a typical day?"

■ "What has your experience been with DKA?"

■ "How regular is your menstrual period?"

How to Intervene When You Suspect an Eating Disorder or Disordered Eating

■ Identify outpatient therapists (e.g., psychologists, social workers, psychiatrists) who are, first of all, experienced in treating eating disorders, and secondly, comfortable treating patients with diabetes and an eating disorder.

- Severe eating disorders, especially anorexia and insulin misuse, are life threatening. Such patients may require hospitalization in an inpatient eating-disorders unit. Identify a psychiatric facility that has experience in the treatment of patients with eating disorders and diabetes.

- It is critical that the patient's diabetes team remains in close contact with providers who specialize in the treatment of eating disorders. Multidisciplinary teamwork and close communication are necessary for effective treatment.

- If it is difficult to locate local outpatient or inpatient resources for your patients with diabetes and eating disorders, contact the state medical society, the state diabetes association, or IAEDP (the International Association of Eating Disorders Professionals Foundation [www.iaedp.com]).

How to Minimize Weight Gain Related to Intensification of Glycemic Control

- Basal-bolus therapy using both glargine and detemir has been associated with less weight gain than therapy using other longer-acting insulins. Physiologic basal-bolus insulin replacement more readily facilitates dieting because mealtime insulin doses can be decreased to adjust for reduced food intake. In addition, there is less need for interprandial snacking than with traditional insulin injection regimens.

- With pump therapy, the patient can manually reduce basal insulin levels during exercise, which will allow him or her to more effectively

continued on page 66

continued from page 65

use exercise to burn off calories without carbohydrate loading beforehand.

Caution regarding pump therapy and eating disorders. Sometimes young women with poor glycemic control due to unrecognized eating disorders and/or insulin omission will be started on insulin pump therapy in the hope of improving glycemic control. This can be dangerous. Unlike other pump patients, who will troubleshoot for insulin nondelivery whenever there is unexplained hyperglycemia, the chronically hyperglycemic individual on a pump will not know when to follow these troubleshooting routines. Therefore, such patients are more prone to develop DKA in the event of pump malfunction or catheter occlusion.

BUILDING MOTIVATION TO CHANGE SELF-CARE BEHAVIOR

The clinician's task in building motivation and overcoming ambivalence about change in self-care behavior is complex and sometimes daunting. There are several considerations in this process, and we will address each in detail.

Different Perspectives about Intensive Therapy

Clinical practice shows us that simply telling patients about the benefits of intensive therapy rarely persuades them to effectively change their self-care behavior. To develop effective communication between provider and patient, there needs to be a convergence of perspectives and goals of treatment. The physician's perspective will often be focused on setting up the treatment plan, i.e., telling the patient what they need to do to improve diabetes control. In general, the clinician's perspective tends to emphasize the benefits of optimizing glycemic control, while undervaluing the extra demands and personal costs required to achieve such control. In contrast, patients often evaluate a new treatment regimen in terms of its immediate costs, demands, and sacrifices and tend to lose sight of the possible future benefits a new therapy may provide. These contrasting perspectives highlight two important considerations.

1. Although improved glycemic control may be the key therapeutic end point, the focus in care should not be exclusively directed at blood glucose management, but should be framed in terms of making diabetes *more manageable.*

2. Treatment methods and rationales should be presented to patients in terms of their own perspective. More specifically, emphasis should be placed on the immediate and direct benefits of intensive therapy, that it provides a *flexible, individualized* treatment program that fits into the demands of daily life.

Uncover Barriers to Intensive Therapy

Some patients have personal barriers that stand in the way of improving diabetes control. Helping patients identify and overcome these hurdles will be a critical task in promoting improved glycemic control. Some of the more common barriers encountered in clinical practice are addressed from a patient-centered viewpoint in the second section of this book, "For the Young Adult: Preparing for Your Journey."

ADDRESS THE PATIENT, NOT THE CLINICAL PRACTICE RECOMMENDATIONS

These two reflections on patient-provider perspectives are helpful. They address one clinical principle (i.e., optimal blood glucose control through intensive therapy) through two lenses for the patient: *1)* your diabetes will become more manageable now and in the future and *2)* intensive therapy will not become an obstacle in your normal, daily life.

Visually, the process of addressing different perspectives will look something like this.

Focus on more immediate benefits to…

↓

Overcome ambivalence about change, which leads to…

↓

Engagement in self-care, which ultimately results in…

↓

Improvement in glycemic control.

Misconceptions that equate intensive diabetes control with intensive self-control. Explaining to the patient that every 1% decline in A1C is only equivalent to a 35-mg/dl reduction in mean blood glucose levels and is associated with a 35–40% decline in risk for microvascular complications will often help the patient understand that even modest improvements in glycemic control can have a major impact on his or her future health.

Fear of hypoglycemia. Patients who are reluctant to intensify therapy and have a history of severe hypoglycemic reactions may be afraid of hypoglycemia. In many of these cases, hypoglycemic reactions have caused personal embarrassment or triggered interpersonal conflict. Directed questioning may be necessary to uncover this barrier.

Unrealistic expectations and perfectionism. Early experiences with diabetes professionals who set unattainable treatment goals and perfectionist expectations can leave the patient with those same unrealistic strivings. More often than not, such goals lead to frustration and disengagement.

Concerns about weight gain associated with intensification of glycemic control. Misuse of insulin can be an effective weight-loss strategy, and the possibility of intentional underdosing or omission of insulin should be considered if the patient has persistent unexplained suboptimal glycemic control despite intensive diabetes self-management education and follow-up.

Set Realistic Goals

Blood glucose monitoring is a crucial tool in the management of diabetes, and patient glucose records are now a major focus of the interaction between patient and provider. However, clinicians often fail to recognize that patients see their blood glucose and A1C levels as more than just objective measures of glycemic control. For patients, these levels translate into a complex judgment of their individual performance, competence, and self-worth.

Goal setting requires that the clinician differentiate between recommended clinical treatment standards (such as the American Diabetes Association Clinical Practice Recommendations) and the goals that are set for the individual patient. For example, giving the patient an ideal, rather than a realistic, A1C target can be counterproductive. Health care providers run the risk of setting up a patient for failure, frustration, and disengagement from care when he or she promotes goals that are too ambitious and/or ignore the realities of the patient's life (such as the competing priorities faced in college) and the complex difficulties of managing diabetes. In contrast, realistic and attainable goals that are appropriate to the patient's aptitudes, motivation, and stage of development will reinforce self-confidence and feelings of efficacy. As patients achieve realistic goals, they become more assured of their success, leading to future progress.

When setting goals, focus on self-care behavior because these practices directly affect A1C and blood glucose levels. Goals need to be set in collaboration *with* the patient (not *for* the patient), and he or she must be able to relate to the goal on a practical level. For example, patients who are athletic will easily relate to the importance of optimizing glycemic control around exercise, and this can be a starting point for engaging them to improve their self-care.

During some of the transitions of the young-adult period, even the most meticulous patients will have difficulty giving diabetes high priority, so practical and realistic expectations are critical to treatment success. Being practical will also minimize the risk that a young adult will become frustrated or burned out. Remind patients and parents that the young-adult period is transitory and dynamic, so difficulties with the diabetes regimen (within reason) are more or less normal and do not indicate a patient's personal failure.

Minimize Performance Pressure

Minimizing performance pressure can be a key element in reducing the chances of diabetes burnout and keeping the patient focused on optimizing his or her diabetes control. The health care provider can reduce performance pressure by

- helping the patient appreciate that blood glucose monitoring is a tool (e.g., a *compass*) to direct diabetes management, rather than a performance measure (e.g., a *test*).

- individualizing blood glucose and glycohemoglobin targets rather than using ideal or standardized levels.

- describing glucose and glycohemoglobin levels with neutral, nonjudgmental language. Use words like "high" or "out of range" instead of "poor" or "bad."

RECOGNIZE THE IMPACT OF CHANGING FAMILIAL AND SOCIAL RELATIONSHIPS

Relationships within the Family

The usually abrupt transfer to personal independence and responsibility for self-care that occurs when young adults with diabetes leave home can be unsettling for both them and their parents.

- The developmental maturity of the young adult must be considered while deciding when to transfer care from the pediatrician to an adult-care provider. Some patients may become overwhelmed by the changes and demands of the early young-adult years. These competing demands sometimes distract the patient from forging ties with a new physician. A young adult who is facing a difficult adjustment to college and has strong bonds with his or her pediatric team may do better if the transfer to adult care is delayed until a later date.

■ The health care provider needs to be attuned to the anxieties that parents may develop as their child gains more independence. Some parents become concerned at the possible consequences of their diminishing role in the young adult's diabetes care. Anxious parents who are overly intrusive and controlling can trigger a destructive cycle of *miscarried helping* (see below) that undermines their child's self-confidence and motivation.

HOW TO PREVENT MISCARRIED HELPING AND TEACH PARENTS POSITIVE INVOLVEMENT

1. Encourage the young-adult patient to bring a parent to an education and updating session. The entire session should be conducted in the presence of the young adult, showing that the patient is the primary focus of the meeting.

2. Listen to the parent's fears, worries, and experiences with previous diabetes providers. Reassure the parents that your goal is to engage their child in diabetes self-care in a way that will optimize current

and future health and to make sure that he or she has regular exams.

3. Emphasize that as a provider you will only speak with the parent when you have the young adult's permission. This includes when both parties are present.

4. Demonstrate positive helping by directly asking your patient how and when his or her parents could be of help.

5. During the first phase of the young-adult period, when the young adult copes with multiple distractions, educate the patient and family to have realistic and appropriate expectations concerning the young adult's blood glucose levels and self-care behaviors.

RECOMMENDATION

If the young adult has had a negative socialization experience growing up with diabetes and does not have a solid, constructive relationship with pediatric care providers, early transfer to an adult provider who has experience with adolescents and young adults with type 1 diabetes is probably in the patient's best interest.

Other Social Relationships

The health care provider also needs to be attuned to the interaction between diabetes and the developing social relationships of the young adult.

■ Misunderstandings of the behavioral changes that occur with unrecognized hypoglycemia are common and can disrupt relationships. Other issues, such as unrealistic expectations and blame, can sabotage relationships and undermine self-care. Inviting partners to participate in medical visits can help uncover these problems.

■ The period when the young-adult patient starts to develop long-term relationships and plans for the future will often signal a stage of receptiveness to improving self-care. Life partners can become influential agents for change, and it is often important to engage them in discussions about treatment options and plans.

RECOGNIZE YOUR IMPACT ON THE PATIENT'S MENTAL HEALTH

Health care providers have an important role in fostering the mental health of a patient with diabetes. Depression, lack of motivation, and disengagement from medical care can be the unintended consequences of the interaction between the patient and health professional.

The positive message of the DCCT and other intervention studies that have established the causal link between glycemic control and the vascular complications of diabetes is that individuals with diabetes have some control over their destiny. However, patients will often perceive another message in the causal link between blood glucose levels and self-care practices—they are to blame for their complications. It is often overlooked that, as evidenced by the data showing that some individuals with relatively low A1C levels develop complications, whereas others with poorer control seem to be protected, hyperglycemia is not the only pathogenic factor in the development of complications.

Many patients with diabetes live with the burden of fear and anxiety about complications and disability, fear and anxiety that is often unwittingly reinforced by health professionals. Complications do not escape mention in educational materials on diabetes or during educational sessions, and few patients need to be reminded of the consequences of neglecting their self-care. There is no evidence that espousing fear successfully motivates patients. On the contrary, if the interaction with the health professional heightens the patient's fears and anxieties, withdrawal from follow-up and self-care are often the unfortunate result.

Sources

ACE Inhibitors in Diabetic Nephropathy Trialist Group: Should all patients with type 1 diabetes mellitus and microalbuminuria receive angiotensin-converting enzyme inhibitors? A meta-analysis of individual patient data. *Ann Intern Med* 134:370–379, 2001

Ahfield JE, Soler NG, Marcus SD: The young adult with diabetes: impact of the disease on marriage and having children. *Diabetes Care* 8:52–56, 1985

American Diabetes Association: *American Diabetes Association Complete Guide to Diabetes.* 4th ed. Alexandria, VA, American Diabetes Association, 2005

American Diabetes Association: Preconception care of women with diabetes (Position Statement). *Diabetes Care* 27 (Suppl. 1):S76–S78, 2004

American Diabetes Association: Preventive foot care in diabetes (Position Statement). *Diabetes Care* 27 (Suppl. 1):S63–S64, 2004

Arnett JJ: Emerging adulthood: a theory of development from the late teens through the twenties. *Am Psychol* 55:469–480, 2000

Anderson BJ, Coyne JC: "Miscarried helping" in the interactions between chronically ill children and their parents. In *Advances in Child Health Psychology*. Johnson JH, Johnson SB, Eds. Gainesville, FL, University of Florida Press, 1991, p. 167–177

Anderson BJ, Mansfield AK: Psychological issues in the treatment of diabetes. In *Joslin's Diabetes Deskbook*. Beaser RS, Ed. Boston, MA, Joslin Diabetes Center, 2001, p. 559–579

Anderson RM: Patient empowerment and the traditional medical model: a case of irreconcilable differences? *Diabetes Care* 18:412–415, 1995

Barbero GJ: Leaving the pediatrician for the internist. *Ann Intern Med* 96:673–674, 1982

Baron RA: Negative effects of destructive criticism: impact on conflict, self-efficacy, and task performance. *J Appl Psychol* 73:199–207, 1988

Betts PR, Jefferson IG, Swift PG: Diabetes care in childhood and adolescence. *Diabet Med* 19 (Suppl 4):61–65, 2002

Bolderman KM: *Putting Your Patients on the Pump*. Alexandria, VA, American Diabetes Association, 2002

Boyle MP, Farukhi Z, Nosky ML: Strategies for improving transition to adult cystic fibrosis care, based on patient and parent views. *Pediatr Pulmonol* 32:428–436, 2001

Bryden KS, Peveler RC, Stein A, Neil A, Mayou RA, Dunger DB: Clinical and psychological course of diabetes from adolescence to young adulthood: a longitudinal cohort study. *Diabetes Care* 24:1536–1540, 2001

Bryden KS, Dunger DB, Mayou RA, Peveler RC, Neil HAW: Poor prognosis of young adults with type 1 diabetes: a longitudinal study. *Diabetes Care* 26:1052–1057, 2003

Clement S: Diabetes self-management education. *Diabetes Care* 18:1204–1214, 1995

DAFNE Study Group: Training in flexible, intensive insulin manage-
ment to enable dietary freedom in people with type 1 diabetes: Dosage Adjustment For Normal Eating (DAFNE) randomised controlled trial. *BMJ* 325:746–751, 2002

Diabetes Control and Complications Trial Research Group: The effect of intensive treatment of diabetes on the development and progression of the long-term complications in insulin-dependent diabetes mellitus. *N Engl J Med* 329:977–986, 1993

el-Hashimy M, Angelico MC, Martin BC, Krolewski AS, Warram JH: Factors modifying the risk of IDDM in offspring of an IDDM parent. *Diabetes* 44:295–299, 1995

Erikson E: *Childhood and Society*. 2nd ed. New York, Norton, 1963

Fairburn CG, Peveler RC, Davies B, Mann JI, Mayou RA: Eating disorders in young adults with insulin dependent diabetes mellitus: a controlled study. *BMJ* 303:17–20, 1991

Goebel-Fabbri AE: Detecting and treating eating disorders in young women with type 1 diabetes. In *Practical Psychology for Diabetes Clinicians*. 2nd ed. Anderson BJ, Rubin RR, Eds. Alexandria, VA, American Diabetes Association, 2002, p. 239–247

Gonder-Frederick LA, Cox DJ, Clarke WL: Helping patients understand, recognize, and avoid hypoglycemia. In *Practical Psychology for Diabetes Clinicians*. 2nd ed. Anderson BJ, Rubin RR, Eds. Alexandria, VA, American Diabetes Association, 2002, p. 113–124

Greenfield S, Kaplan SH, Ware JE Jr, Yano EM, Frank HJ: Patients' participation in medical care: effects on blood sugar control and quality of life in diabetes. *J Gen Intern Med* 3:448–457, 1988

Haire-Joshu D, Glasgow RE, Tibbs TL: Smoking and diabetes (Technical Review). *Diabetes Care* 22:1887–1898, 1999

Herman WH: Clinical evidence: glycaemic control in diabetes. *BMJ* 319:104–106, 1999

Holzmeister LA: *Diabetes Carbohydrate and Fat Gram Guide*. 3rd ed. Alexandria, VA, American Diabetes Association, 2005

Hovind P, Tarnow L, Rossing K, Rossing P, Eising S, Larsen N, Binder C, Parving HH: Decreasing incidence of severe diabetic microangiopathy in type 1 diabetes. *Diabetes Care* 26:1258–1264, 2003

Johnston-Brooks CH, Lewis MA, Garg G: Self-efficacy impacts self-care and HbA1c in young adults with type 1 diabetes. *Psychosom Med* 64:43–51, 2002

Jones JM, Lawson ML, Daneman D, Olmsted MP, Rodin G: Eating disorders in adolescent females with and without type 1 diabetes: cross-sectional study. *BMJ* 320:1563–1566, 2000

Kaplan SH, Greenfield S, Ware JE: Assessing the effects of the physician-patient interactions on the outcomes of chronic disease. *Med Care* 27 (Suppl. 3):S110–S127, 1989

Kaufman F, Halvorson MJ, Lohry J: *Putting Your Diabetes on the Pump*. Alexandria, VA, American Diabetes Association, 2001

Kipps S, Bahu T, Ong K, Ackland FM, Brown RS, Fox CT, Griffin NK, Knight AH, Mann NP, Neil HA, Simpson H, Edge JA, Dunger DB: Current methods of transfer of young people with type 1 diabetes to adult services. *Diabet Med* 19:649–650, 2002

Krolewski AS, Warram JH, Christlieb AR, Busick EJ, Kahn CR: The changing history of nephropathy in type 1 diabetes. *Am J Med* 78:785–794, 1985

Levinson DJ, Darrow CN, Klein EB, Levinson MH, McKee B: *The Seasons of a Man's Life*. New York, Knopf, 1978

Lorenzen T, Pociot F, Stilgren L, Kristiansen OP, Johannesen J, Olsen PB, Walmar A, Larsen A, Albrechtsen NC, Eskildsen PC, Andersen OO, Nerup J: Predictors of IDDM recurrence in offspring of Danish IDDM patients. *Diabetologia* 41:666–673, 1998

Mathiesen ER, Hommel E, Hansen HP, Smidt UM, Parving H-H: Randomised controlled trial of long term efficacy of captopril on preservation of kidney function in normotensive patients with insulin dependent diabetes and microalbuminuria. *BMJ* 319:24–25, 1999

McCulloch DK, Glasgow RE, Hampson SE, Wagner E: A systematic approach to diabetes management in the post-DCCT era. *Diabetes Care* 17:765–769, 1994

Mellinger DC: Preparing students with diabetes for life at college. *Diabetes Care* 26:2675–2678, 2003

Orr DP, Fineberg NS, Gay DL: Glycemic control and transfer of health care among adolescents with insulin dependent diabetes mellitus. *J Adolesc Health* 18:44–47, 1996

Perkins BA, Ficociello LH, Silva KH, Finkelstein DM, Warram JH, Krolewski AS: Regression of microalbuminuria in type 1 diabetes. *N Engl J Med* 348:2285–2293, 2003

Peveler RC, Davies BA, Mayou RA, Fairburn CG, Mann JI: Self-care behaviour and blood glucose control in young adults with type 1 diabetes mellitus. *Diabet Med* 10:74–80, 1993

Peveler RC, Bryden KS, Neil HAW, Fairburn CG, Mayou RA, Dunger DB, Turner HM: The relationship of disordered eating habits and attitudes to clinical outcomes in young adult females with type 1 diabetes. *Diabetes Care* 28:84–88, 2005

Polonsky WH: *Diabetes Burnout: What To Do When You Can't Take It Anymore.* Alexandria, VA, American Diabetes Association, 1999

Polonsky WH, Anderson BJ, Lohrer PA, Aponte JE, Jacobson AM, Cole CF: Insulin omission in women with IDDM. *Diabetes Care* 17:1178–1185, 1994

Polonsky WH, Anderson BJ, Lohrer PA, Welch G, Jacobson AM, Aponte JE, Schwartz CE: Assessment of diabetes-related distress. *Diabetes Care* 18:754–760, 1995

Reiss J, Gibson R: Health care transition: destinations unknown. *Pediatrics* 110:1307–1314, 2002

Rollnick S, Kinnersley P, Stott N: Methods of helping patients with behaviour change. *BMJ* 307:188–190, 1993

Rollnick S, Mason P, Butler C: *Health Behavior Change: A Guide for Practitioners.* Edinburgh, U.K., Churchill Livingstone, 1999

Rosenstock J, Schwartz SL, Clark CM, Park GD, Donley DW, Edwards MB: Basal insulin therapy in type 2 diabetes: 28-week comparison of insulin glargine (HOE 901) and NPH insulin. *Diabetes Care* 24:631–636, 2001

Rydall AC, Rodin GM, Olmsted M, Devenyi RG, Daneman D: Disordered eating behavior and microvascular complications in young women with insulin-dependent diabetes mellitus. *N Engl J Med* 336:1849–1854, 1997

Sawyer SM, Blair S, Bowes G: Chronic illness in adolescents: transfer or transition to adult services? *J Paediatr Child Health* 33:88–90, 1997

Selkowitz Litt A: *The College Student's Guide to Eating Well on Campus.* Bethesda, MD, Tulip Hill Press, 2005

UK Prospective Diabetes Study Group: Tight blood pressure control and risk of macrovascular and microvascular complications in type 2 diabetes: UKPDS 38. *BMJ* 317:703–713, 1998

Vague P, Selam JL, Skeie S, De Leeuw I, Elte JW, Haahr H, Kristensen A, Draeger E: Insulin detemir is associated with more predictable glycemic control and reduced risk of hypoglycemia than NPH insulin in patients with type 1 diabetes on a basal-bolus regimen with premeal insulin aspart. *Diabetes Care* 26:590–596, 2003

Vinicor F: Barriers to translation of the Diabetes Control and Complications Trial. *Diabetes Reviews* 2:371–383, 1994

Warram JH, Martin BC, Krolewski AS: Risk of IDDM in children of diabetic mothers decreases with increasing maternal age at pregnancy. *Diabetes* 40:1679–1684, 1991

Wechsler H, Wuethrich B: *Dying to Drink: Confronting Binge Drinking on College Campuses.* Emmaus, PA, Rodale Books, 2002

Weissberg-Benchell J, Antisdel-Lomaglio J, Seshadri R: Insulin pump therapy: a meta-analysis. *Diabetes Care* 26:1079–1087, 2003

Welch GW, Jacobson AM, Polonsky W: The Problem Areas in Diabetes (PAID) Scale: an examination of its clinical utility. *Diabetes Care* 20:760–766, 1997

White NH, Cleary PA, Dahms W, Goldstein D, Malone J, Tamborlane WV, Diabetes Control and Complications Trial (DCCT)/ Epidemiology of Diabetes Interventions and Complications (EDIC) Research Group: Beneficial effects of intensive therapy of diabetes during adolescence: outcomes after conclusion of the Diabetes Control and Complications Trial (DCCT). *J Pediatr* 139:804–812, 2001

Williams GC, Freedman ZR, Deci EL: Supporting autonomy to motivate patients with diabetes for glucose control. *Diabetes Care* 21:1644–1651, 1998

Winocour PH: Effective diabetes care: a need for realistic targets. *BMJ* 324:1577–1580, 2002

Wolpert HA: *Smart Pumping.* Alexandria, VA, American Diabetes Association, 2002

Wolpert HA: Working with young adults who have type 1 diabetes. In *Practical Psychology for Diabetes Clinicians*. 2nd ed. Anderson BJ, Rubin RR, Eds. Alexandria, VA, American Diabetes Association, 2002, p. 161–169

Wolpert HA, Anderson BJ: Management of diabetes: are doctors framing the benefits from the wrong perspective? *BMJ* 323:994–996, 2001

Wolpert HA, Anderson BJ: Metabolic control matters: why is the message lost in the translation? The need for realistic goal-setting in diabetes care. *Diabetes Care* 24:1301–1303, 2001

Wolpert HA, Anderson BJ: Young adults with diabetes: need for a new treatment paradigm. *Diabetes Care* 24:1513–1514, 2001

Writing Team for the Diabetes Control and Complications Trial/Epidemiology of Diabetes Interventions and Complications Research Group: Effect of intensive therapy on the microvascular complications of type 1 diabetes mellitus. *JAMA* 287:2563–2569, 2002

Wysocki T: Graduating to adult care. *Diabetes Self-Management* 11:41–43, 1994

Wysocki T, Hough BS, Ward KM, Green LB: Diabetes mellitus in the transition to adulthood: adjustment, self-care, and health care status. *J Dev Behav Pediatr* 13:194–201, 1992

Zhang L, Krzentowski G, Albert A, Lefebvre PJ: Risk of developing retinopathy in Diabetes Control and Complications Trial type 1 diabetic patients with good or poor metabolic control. *Diabetes Care* 24:1275–1279, 2001

About the American Diabetes Association

The American Diabetes Association is the nation's leading voluntary health organization supporting diabetes research, information, and advocacy. Its mission is to prevent and cure diabetes and to improve the lives of all people affected by diabetes. The American Diabetes Association is the leading publisher of comprehensive diabetes information. Its huge library of practical and authoritative books for people with diabetes covers every aspect of self-care—cooking and nutrition, fitness, weight control, medications, complications, emotional issues, and general self-care.

To order American Diabetes Association books: Call 1-800-232-6733. Or log on to http://store.diabetes.org

To join the American Diabetes Association: Call 1-800-806-7801. www.diabetes.org/membership

For more information about diabetes or ADA programs and services: Call 1-800-342-2383. E-mail: AskADA@diabetes.org or log on to www.diabetes.org

To locate an ADA/NCQA Recognized Provider of quality diabetes care in your area: www.ncqa.org/dprp

To find an ADA Recognized Education Program in your area: Call 1-888-232-0822. www.diabetes.org/recognition/education.asp

To join the fight to increase funding for diabetes research, end discrimination, and improve insurance coverage: Call 1-800-342-2383. www.diabetes.org/advocacy

To find out how you can get involved with the programs in your community: Call 1-800-342-2383. See below for program Web addresses.

American Diabetes Month: educational activities aimed at those diagnosed with diabetes—month of November. www.diabetes.org/ADM

American Diabetes Alert: annual public awareness campaign to find the undiagnosed—held the fourth Tuesday in March. www.diabetes.org/alert

The Diabetes Assistance & Resources Program (DAR): diabetes awareness program targeted to the Latino community. www.diabetes.org/DAR

African American Program: diabetes awareness program targeted to the African American community. www.diabetes.org/africanamerican

Awakening the Spirit: Pathways to Diabetes Prevention & Control: diabetes awareness program targeted to the Native American community. www.diabetes.org/awakening

To find out about an important research project regarding type 2 diabetes: www.diabetes.org/ada/research.asp

To obtain information on making a planned gift or charitable bequest: Call 1-888-700-7029. www.diabetes.org/ada/plan.asp

To make a donation or memorial contribution: Call 1-800-342-2383. www.diabetes.org/ada/cont.asp